YOUR KNOWLEDGE HAS VALUE

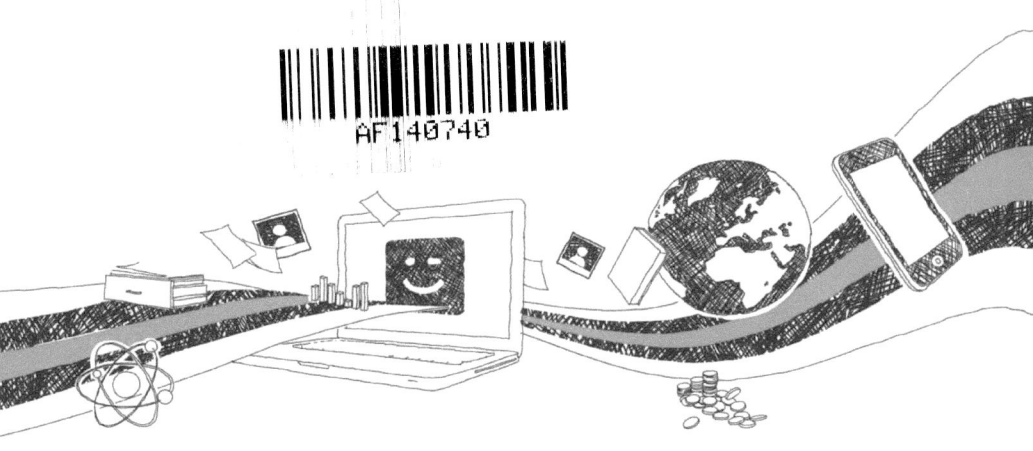

AF140740

- We will publish your bachelor's and
  master's thesis, essays and papers

- Your own eBook and book -
  sold worldwide in all relevant shops

- Earn money with each sale

Upload your text at www.GRIN.com
and publish for free

GRIN ☺

Bibliographic information published by the German National Library:

The German National Library lists this publication in the National Bibliography; detailed bibliographic data are available on the Internet at http://dnb.dnb.de .

This book is copyright material and must not be copied, reproduced, transferred, distributed, leased, licensed or publicly performed or used in any way except as specifically permitted in writing by the publishers, as allowed under the terms and conditions under which it was purchased or as strictly permitted by applicable copyright law. Any unauthorized distribution or use of this text may be a direct infringement of the author s and publisher s rights and those responsible may be liable in law accordingly.

Imprint:

Copyright © 2017 GRIN Verlag
Print and binding: Books on Demand GmbH, Norderstedt Germany
ISBN: 9783668596948

This book at GRIN:

https://www.grin.com/document/384386

Buli Tadese

The Production Performance of the Ethiopian Indigenous Chickens

GRIN Verlag

GRIN - Your knowledge has value

Since its foundation in 1998, GRIN has specialized in publishing academic texts by students, college teachers and other academics as e-book and printed book. The website www.grin.com is an ideal platform for presenting term papers, final papers, scientific essays, dissertations and specialist books.

Visit us on the internet:

http://www.grin.com/

http://www.facebook.com/grincom

http://www.twitter.com/grin_com

JIMMA UNIVERSY COLLEGE OF AGRICULTUR

AND

VETERNERYMEDICE

DEPARTMENT OF ANIMAL SCIENCE

(ANIMAL PRODUCTION, MSC)

REVIEW ON:-

PRODUCTION PERFORMANCE OF ETHIOPI INDIGENIOUSE CHICKEN

BY: - BULI TADESE WAYESA

December, 2017, ETHIOPIA.

Table of Contents

List of Tables

ABSTRACT

Indigenous village chicken is the most prominent class of livestock in the country and constitutes about 60-80% of the total poultry population, their productivity is low because of poor nutrition and low genetic potential. The number of flock per household in most Ethiopian communities is small constituting on average of 7–10 mature chickens 20–24 adult hens, a male birds (cock) and a number of growers of varies ages. Such production system may result in slow growth and poor layers of small sized eggs. About 40-60% of the chicks hatched die during the first 8 weeks of age mainly due to disease and predators attack. About half of the eggs produced have to be hatched to replace chicken that have died and the brooding time of the laying hens is longer, with many brooding cycles required to compensate for its unsuccessful brooding. Pullets and cockerels reached sexual maturity at an average age of 6.4 months and 5.7 months, respectively. Even though the productivity of local chicken is very poor, they are very important to withstand certain harsh environmental conditions, and can perform better under poor management than cross and exotic breeds, they are also well known to possess desirable characters such as ideal mother, good sister, hatch their own eggs, excellent foragers, resistance to common poultry disease and special meat and egg quality (flavor), hard egg shells

1. Introduction

Animal production in general and chicken production in particular plays important socio- economic roles in developing countries (Alders, 2004). The Ethiopian indigenous chickens are none descriptive breeds closely related to the Jungle fowl and vary in color, comb type, body conformation and weight and may or may not possess shank feather. According to CSA, 2013, the total chicken population in the country is estimated to be 51.35 million of which (96.83%) are indigenous chickens, indicating the significance of local chickens as potential resource of the country.

The total chicken egg and meat production in Ethiopia is also estimated to be about 78,000 and 72,300 metric tons, respectively from which more than 90% of the national chicken meat and egg output is contributed by local chickens. They are characterized by slow growth, late maturity and low production performance .According to Aboe *et al.* (2006), although indigenous village chicken is the most prominent class of livestock in the country and constitutes about 60-80% of the total poultry population, their productivity is low because of poor nutrition and low genetic potential. The mean annual egg production of indigenous chickens is estimated at 60 small eggs with thick shell and deep yellow yolk color (Yami and Dessie, 1997). Provision of animal protein, generation of extra cash incomes and religious/cultural considerations are amongst the major reasons for keeping village chickens by rural communities (Alders *et al.*, 2009). The number of flock per household in most Ethiopian communities is small constituting on average of 7–10 mature chickens 20–24 adult hens, a male birds (cock) and a number of growers of varies ages. Such production system may result in slow growth and poor layers of small sized eggs (Tadellea and Ogle, 2001).

The productivity of local scavenging hens is low, not only because of low egg production potential, but also due to high chick mortality. About 40 60% of the chicks hatched die during the first 8 weeks of age (Hoyle, 1992, Dessie 1996 and CACC, 2003) mainly due to disease and predators attack. It is estimated that, under scavenging conditions, the reproductive cycle consists of 20 day lying phase, 21-day incubation phase and finally a 56-days brooding phase (Yami and Dessie1997). This implies that the number of clutches per hen per year is probably 2-3. Assuming 3 clutches per hen per year, the hen would have to stay for about 168 days out of production every year, entirely engaged in brooding activities.

The low productivity of the indigenous stock could also partially be attributed to the low management standard of the traditional production system. It has been seen that the provision of vaccination, improved feeding, clean water and night time enclosure improves the production performance of the indigenous chickens, but not to an economically acceptable level (Abebe, 1992; Burley, 1957 and Teketel, 1986)

Objective

To Review the productive performance of Ethiopian indigenous chickens.

2.Literature Review

2.1. Poultry production systems

In Ethiopia poultry production systems show a clear distinction between the traditional, low input system on the one hand and modern production systems using relatively advanced technology on the other hand (Alemu, 1995). The traditional poultry production system comprises of the indigenous chickens and characterized by small flock size, low input and output and periodic devastation of the flock by disease. There is no separate poultry house and the chickens live in family dwellings together with human beings. It is by natural incubation and brooding that chicks are hatched and raised all over the rural Ethiopia. A broody hen hatching, rearing and protecting few number of chicks (6-8) ceases egg laying during the entire incubation and brooding periods of 77 days. Yet the successes of the hatching and brooding process depends on the maternal instinct of the broody hen and prevalence of predators in the area, such as birds of prey, pets and some wild animals, all of which are listed as the major causes of premature death of chicks in Ethiopia (Solomon 2007).

2.2 Production Performance of Indigenous chicken

The productive performance of indigenous scavenging chickens of Ethiopia is low because of their low egg production potential, high chicken mortality and longer reproductive cycle (slow growth rate, late sexual maturity and broodiness for extended period (Besbes, 2009). Pullets and cockerels reached sexual maturity at an average age of 6.4 months and 5.7 months, respectively. Even though the productivity of local chicken is very poor, they are very important to withstand certain harsh environmental conditions, and can perform better under poor management than cross and exotic breeds, they are also well known to possess desirable characters such as ideal mother, good sister, hatch their own eggs, excellent foragers, resistance to common poultry disease and special meat and egg quality (flavor), hard egg shells (Abdelqader *et al.*, 2007). The low productivity of the indigenous stock could also partially be attributed to the low management standard of the traditional household poultry production system. It have been seen that the provision of vaccination, improved feeding , clean water and night time enclosure improve the performance of the indigenous chickens(; and Abebe, 1992 and Solomon 2007).

In Ethiopia Indigenous chickens are the most wide spread and almost every rural family owners of chickens, which provide a valuable source of family protein and income (Tadelle *et al.*, 2003). Traditional free scavenging is the common production system (no adequate supply of feeding, housing and health care). This production system results poor productive performance of indigenous chickens (low egg production performance, small sized egg, long sexual maturity of hens and cockerels, high chicken mortality and chickens were exposed to predators). Because of non- genetic factors such as feeding, housing and health care and other management practices have a much greater impact on production than genetics under scavenging system of production.

According to Adem and Teshome,(2016), the hatchability percentage of local chicken showed in the study area was 80%. This result was higher as compared to the value of 70% reported by Solomon (2007) and 59.6% reported by Melkamu and Andarge (2013). The higher percentage observed due to small number of eggs sited per hen for hatching and preparation of good sitting material prior to incubation. This might be an indication of good fertility and brooding of indigenous chickens (Adem Abegaz and Teshome,(2016).

Table 1.Summary of Production performance of local chicken in different study area .

Item	Adem and Teshome ,(2016)	MELAKU TAREKE ADAL(2016).	Mogesetal. (2010)	CACC 2003 and Alemu Yami 19970
Average age of cockerels at 1st mating (months)	5.33	5.86	24.6	-
Average age of local pullets at 1 stegg (months)	6.8	5.87	27.5	6
Average number of eggs/hen per clutch	14	12.81	15.7	12
Number of clutches/hen per year		3.45	3.83	4
Average egg production/hen per year	56	53.18	60	60
Average Egg Weight(gm)	40			38
Average number of Egg set for hatching(No.)	10	13.59	13	
Average number of chick hatch edfrom seted egg(No.)	8	8.81	11	
Hatchability %	80	64.85	82.6	70

Source Summery from Review

Local chickens are appropriate under the traditional production system with low input levels, that makes the best use of locally available resources and hatch their eggs and brood chicks which are important traits under the present Ethiopian conditions (Yami and Dessie, 1997 and (Solomon,2007). The total national annual poultry meat and eggs production were estimated at 72 ,300 and 78 ,000 metric tons, respectively, Resulting in per capita consumption of 57 eggs and 2.85 kg of poultry meat.

Table 2. Productivity indicators of the traditional, poultry production systems in Ethiopia.

Item	Traditional (indigenous)	Breeding centers	Commercial farms
Average egg weight(g	38	56	56
Mean laying period/ hen(days)	20	>200	>200
Eggs/hen per year	60	200	230
Natural incubation period (days)	21	NA	NA
Natural brooding period (days)	56	NA	NA
Mean total days of out of laying	96	NA	NA
Chick mortality (%)	40	5-10	5-6
Fertility (%)	75	80	90
Hatchability (%)	70	65	80
Age at first egg(days)	180	150	145
Slaughter weight at 12 months	1.5	NA	NA
Mortality of adult flock (%)	20-30	6-8	5-6
Mortality of broilers (%)	NA	NA	10-15
Slaughter weight at 8 weeks(kg)	NA	NA	1.8
Adult weight (kg)	1.5	NA	NA

Source: CACC 2003 and Alemu 1997 cited by Solomon, 2007

2.2.1 Flock performance

The indigenous chickens attain their sexual maturity of laying eggs at averages of 6.8 months (Adem and Teshome,2016)and 7-8 months which reported by Mogesses (2007) and later than 6.33 month's which was reported by Meseret (2010). The average body weight of 0.914 kg at first lay was 42% lower than the average body weight of 1.3 kg (Fisseha Moges et al., 2010). This might be associated with differences in the breed of chicken and other factors related to feeding and management of chicken. The delayed sexual maturity for laying egg of local chickens might be as a result of: poor management and Absence of intensive management system and selection among local chickens (Adem A and Teshome, 2016). Productivity of birds was related to agricultural calendar and age of birds. Higher egg production is always expected at the time of land preparation, sowing and during and after harvesting. Pullets produce higher number of eggs in their first year of production than in the subsequent year(s).

2.2.2. Egg production performances

The egg production potential of local chicken is 30-60 eggs year/hen with an average of 38 g egg weight under village management conditions in Ethiopia. With this potential of indigenous chicken, the demand of egg and chicken meat of Ethiopian populations cannot be satisfied (Geleta *et al.*, 2013). According to the study by the Ministry of Agriculture (1980), average annual egg production of the native chicken is estimated to be 30 – 40 eggs/ hen/year under village conditions and this could be increased to 80 eggs/hen/year with the provision of improved feeding, housing and health care. Even though, Solomon (2003b) reported that average annual egg production of the native chicken was 40-60 eggs under village condition and this could be improved to 80-100 eggs on station. Testing the response of the indigenous chicken under good housing, feeding and management increase in the productive performance of indigenous chicken with improved environment and management but not to an economically acceptable level (Solomon, 2003b).

According to Nebiyu et al, (2013), the average age at first lay of village chickens 6.5 months higher than the average age at first lay of 6.33 months (Meseret Molla, 2010). The average body weight of 0.914 kg at first lay in the present study was 42% lower than the average body weight of 1.3 kg (Fisseha Moges et al., 2010). This might be associated with differences in the breed of chicken and other factors related to feeding and management of chicken. The mean egg weight of 39.4 g in the present study was 3.4% higher than the mean egg weight of 38.1 g (Njenga, 2005). On the other hand, the mean egg weight in the present study was 13.7% lower than the mean egg weight of 44.8 g (Bogale , 2008) and 8.6% lower than the mean egg weight 42.9 g (Halima, 2007).

Indigenous flocks are considered to be very poor in egg production performance attributed to low genetic potential, poor management and long natural reproductive cycle. It is estimated that, under scavenging conditions, the reproductive cycle of indigenous hens consists of 20-days of laying phase, 21-days of incubation phase and 56-days of brooding phase (Alemu and Tadelle, 1997).Also From the report of CSA (2011), the average length egg-laying period/hen was also determined in breeds and environmental managements systems of which estimated numbers indigenous chicken 21 days of incubation phases.

The egg production of local layers increased by 15% as a result of supplementation with a daily ration of 60 g/head. This result also agrees   with Alemu and Tadelle (1997) who reported that there is an increase in the egg production performance of local hens with improvement in nutritional status, but not to an economically acceptable level. The mean total egg mass of local layers kept under household conditions was 1.5 kg /hen. Thus there seems to be no economic justification for supplementary feeding of scavenging local layers due to their poor feed utilization efficiencies.

2.2.3. Meat production performance

The meat production ability of local stocks is also limited compared to the exotic birds. Local males may reach 1.5 kg live weight at 6 months of age and females about 30% less. The carcass weight of local stocks at 6 month of age was 550 gram which was significantly lower than that of White Leghorn (875gm). Tadelle (2003) reported that males are 36 percent heavier than their female contemporaries at 18 weeks of age. According to Tadelle (1996) the overall mean live weight of local hens in three different altitudes of the central highlands of Ethiopia were 1129.8 + 59 (ranging from 999 to 1282), with birds at high altitude being heaviest which is probably related to increased availability of feed resources in the immediate environment as the villagers produce more cereals and grow two crops per year and smaller flock size. The chicken meat consumption in Ethiopia as pointed out by Sonaiya (1990), in recent years; rural poultry have assumed a much greater role as suppliers of animal protein for both rural and urban dwellers. This is because of the recurrent droughts, disease and decreased grazing land, which have resulted in significantly reduced supplies of meat from cattle, sheep and goats. Poultry is the only affordable species to be slaughtered at home by resource-poor farmers, as the prices of other species are too high, and have increased substantially in recent years.

According to Alemu (1987) the per capita consumption was about 2.85 kg of chicken meat per annum in Ethiopia, which are very low figures by international standards. Poultry meat is relatively cheap and affordable sources of protein for most consumers compared to other animal products such as beef. Muchenje et al. (2001) reported that poultry provide major opportunities for increased protein production and incomes for smallholder farmers. Village chicken in Ethiopia provides 12.5 kg of poultry meat per capital per year, whereas cattle provide only 5.34 kg" (Kitalyi, 1997). FAO (2010) reported that the human population benefits greatly from poultry meat and eggs, which provide food containing high-quality protein, and a low level of fat with a desirable fatty acid profiles. To improve chicken production and to satisfy the demands of protein foods, participation of family members in the household is highly required in the phenomena of poultry productions.

Table 3: African human population and poultry meat consumption.

Country	Human Population				Poultry Meat Consumption Kg/Person/year		
	2000	2010	2015	2020	2000	2007	2009
Ethiopia	65.6	83	92	101.1	0.6	0.6	0.6
Egypt	67.7	81.1	88.2	94.8	8.6	10.5	10
Kenya	31.3	40.5	46.3	52.6	0.4	0.6	0.6
Nigeria	123.7	158.4	179.8	203.9	1.3	1.7	1.7
Somalia	7.4	9.3	10.6	12.2	-	-	-
Togo	4.8	6	6.7	7.3	4.1	4.4	6
Uganda	24.2	33.4	39.1	45.4	1.8	1.4	1.4

Source:http://www.thepoultrysite.com/articles/2973/global-poultry-trends-2013-continued-upward-trend-inchicken-consumption-in-africa-and-oceania/.

2.2.4. Breaking broodiness

Broodiness is a vital characteristic of traditionally managed local birds and the physiological mechanism is a prerequisite to sustain the present system at least until local farmers start to use other means of incubation. Normally, once a bird becomes broody and is not used for hatching eggs, she will remain broody for 3-4 weeks. Traditionally, households attempts to increase egg production by stimulating broody birds to resume egg lying. The basis for these practices is to disturb the broody bird and to cause a hormonal shift so that it starts to lay eggs again within 8 -10 days. Because of this human interference, the number of clutches and eggs produced /year /bird were increased. If the hen hatches eggs it will stay with its brood for up to eight weeks. Some farmers, set eggs under two birds at the same time, and after hatching give all the chicks to one of the hens. However, regular stimulation of birds to resume egg laying as a measure taken by households to improve laying performance of hens increases egg production by about 80% and is testimony that chicken ecotypes are shaped not only by the environment but also by human intervention.

The traditional methods of breaking broodiness are disturbing the laying nest (Place some material on egg laying place), and tying the legs of broody hen and hanging of the hen upside down position could break broodiness within 3 to 4 days depending on the degree of strength of broodiness which vary from hen to hen. Also According to Similarly, Dereje (2001), Adele (2003) and Mammo(2006) reported that piercing the nostril with feather, moving the bird to a nearby house for a couple of days and hanging upside down are effective in breaking broodiness within 3 to 4 days .The hens resume laying soon after breaking broodiness resulting in increase in total annual egg production. This result is in agreement with that of Rushton (1996) as cited by Kitalyi (1998) who reported higher egg productivity (143 eggs/hen/year) by the Ethiopia indigenous chickens with the proper management of broody hen. These results also agree with that of Tadelle (1996), Dereje (2001), Tadelle et al. (2003) and Resource-Center (2005) who reported that households traditionally attempt to break broodiness to resume egg lying with final goal of increasing egg productivity.

Table 3. Practices of breaking broodiness in the study area (% of HH)

Practice to break Broodiness	Mid-Highlands	High land	Lowland	Overall
Tying	25.0(8^{NS})	34.5(10^{NS})	29.0(9^{NS})	29.3(27)
Piercing feather in the nose	21.9(7)	13.8(4)	12.9(4)	16,3(15)
Place some material on nose	31.3(10)	27.6(8)	32.3(10)	30.4(28)
Place some materials on egg laying place	15.6(5)	13.8(40	16.1(5)	15.2(14)
Hanging upside down	6.3(2)	10.3930	9.7(3)	8.7(8)
Taking in to neighborhoods	5.8125	6.3448	6.2581	16.587

Source: Matiwos Habte, Negassi Ameha and Solomon Demeke, 2013

2.2.5. Hatchability

The production potential of backyard chickens can only be increased when there are adequate numbers of viable chickens available for replacement of the uneconomical birds. This is mainly a function of the quality of the eggs set for hatching (North, 1984). The higher the proportion of quality eggs, the better hatchability. Backyard chickens are scavengers, and there seems to be a wide variation in their hatching performance compared with commercial poultry. Fargo *et al.* (2000) reported hatchability variation ranging between 63.1 and 84.1% of eggs under backyard conditions. Hatchability is affected by several factors including nutritional and health status, genetic factors and physical, storage and incubation conditions of the eggs (Matiwos Habte, 2012). Seasonal fluctuations could also cause wide variability in hatchability. A prolonged egg holding period may cause deterioration in the interior egg quality and increase the risks of embryonic mortality (Prabakaran *et al.*, 1984). The number of eggs set under a broody hen could also affect hatchability. It is suggested that incubation of a single egg beyond the capacity of broody hen could result in reduction of hatchability by 0.23% (Farooq *et al.*, 2003).

Hatchability and rate of chick survival are one of the major determinant factors of productivity in poultry. Commonly incubate eggs during dry seasons and use '' hammattu'' (clay pot with straw bedding) as an incubation box. A broody hen hatching, rearing and protecting few number of chicks 6 to 8 ceases egg laying during the entire incubation and brooding periods of 81 days. Yet the successes of the hatching and brooding process depends on the maternal instinct of the broody hen and prevalence of predators in the area, such as birds of prey, pets and some wild animals, all of which are listed as the major causes of premature death of chicks in Ethiopia. According to the results of the discussions made with key informants, the number of eggs set per hen depends on availability of eggs, size of eggs and size of broody hen and the maternal instinct of the broody hen. The overall mean number of eggs reported to be 11.32 eggs with minimum of 6 and maximum 20 eggs per hen, the value of which agrees with Sonaiya and Swan (2004), Udo et al (2001).

3. Challenges in traditional chicken production Performance

3.1. Disease and predators'

The most striking problem in traditional chicken production systems is the high mortality rate which could reach as high as 80–90% within the first few weeks after hatching, due to diseases and predation (Wilson *et al.*, 1987), Newcastle disease (NCD) is highly infectious and causes more losses than any other diseases in the tropics. The same author reported 96.4% of village chicken owners had no culture of vaccination against poultry diseases in North West Ethiopia. The disease spreads rapidly through the flock and mortality could reach up to 100% (Nigussie *et al.*, 2003; Serkalem *et al.*, 2005; Nwanta *et al.*, 2008). Among the infectious diseases, NCD, salmonelloses, coccidioses and fowl pox are considered to be the most important causes of mortality in local chicken while predators are an additional causes of loss (Eshetu *et al.*, 2001).

3.2. In adequate Feed Quantity and Quality

The other major limiting factor of traditional or village chicken production is feed, in terms of both quantity and quality (Mohamed and Abate, 1995). The nutritional status of local laying hens from chemical analysis of crop contents indicated that protein was below the requirement for optimum egg production and the deficiency is more serious during the short rainy and dry seasons (Tegene, 1992; Alemu and Tadelle, 1997). In addition to the above mentioned constraints; Singh (1990) reported other vital problems affecting the productivity of traditional or village chicken including: low productivity of local chicken (attributed to low genetic potential, disease and poor chicken management practices and poor extension services.

4. Conclusion

Local chickens play an important role in supplying high quality protein to the family food balance and providing small disposable cash income in addition to the socio-religious functions for people . The productive performance of indigenous scavenging chickens of Ethiopia is low because of their low egg production potential, high chicken mortality and longer reproductive cycle (slow growth rate, late sexual maturity and broodiness for extended period .The low productivity of the indigenous stock could also partially be attributed to the low management standard of the traditional household poultry production system. Higher egg production is always expected at the time of land preparation, sowing and during and after harvesting. In addition, it was understood that pullets produce higher number of eggs in their first year of production than in the subsequent year(s) .The egg production potential of local chicken is 30-60 eggs year/ hen with an average of 38 g egg weight under village management conditions However, regular stimulation of birds to resume egg laying as a measure taken by households to improve laying performance of hens increases egg production by about 80% and is testimony that chicken ecotypes are shaped not only by the environment but also by human intervention.

5. REFERENCES

Abassa, K.P. 1995. Improving food security in Africa: The ignored contribution of live-stock joint ECA/FAO agricultural division.monograph.No.14, Addis Ababa, Ethiopia.

Abdelqader A, Wollny C and Gauly M (2007) Characterization of Local Chicken Production Systems and their Potential Under Different Levels of Management Practices in Jordan. Trop Anim Health Pro 39:155-164.

Aberra, M., S. Maak and G. von Lengerken, 2005. The performance of naked neck and their F1 crosses with Lohmann White and New Hampshire chicken breeds under long-term heat stress conditions. Ethiop. J. Anim. Prod., 5: 91-106.

Abraham, L. and T. Yayneshet, 2010. Performance of exotic and indigenous poultry breeds managed by smallholder farmers in northern Ethiopia. Livestock Res. Rural Dev., Vol. 22.

Chencha Chebo and Hailemikael Nigussie, 2016. Performances, Breeding Practices and Trait Preferences of Local Chicken Ecotypes in Southern Zone of Tigray, Northern Ethiopia. *Asian Journal of Poultry Science, 10: 158-164.*

Halima, H., 2007. Phenotypic and Genetic Characterization of indigenous chicken populations in northwest Ethiopia. PhD thesis submitted to the Faculty of Natural and Agricultural Sciences Department of Animal, Wildlife and Grassland Sciences University of the Free State, Bloemfontein, South Africa.

Mekonnen G/egziabher (2007) Characterization of smallholder poultry production and marketing system of dale, Wonsho and Loka Abaya Weredas of southern EthiopiaM.Sc Thesis, Awassa College of Agriculture, Hawassa University, Hawassa, Ethiopia.

Meseret M (2010) Characterization of village chicken production and marketing system in GommaWereda, Jimma zone, Ethiopia. M.Sc. Thesis, Jimma University, Jimma, Ethiopia.

Samson L, Endalew B (2010) Survey on Village Based Chicken Production and Utilization System in Mid Rift Valley of Oromia, Ethiopia. Adami-Tullu Agricultural Research Center, Poultry Technology Research Team, Ziway, Ethiopia, Global Veterinaria 5: 198-203.

Tadelle D (1996) Studies on village poultry production systems in the central high altitudes of Ethiopia M.Sc Thesis, Swedish University of

YOUR KNOWLEDGE HAS VALUE

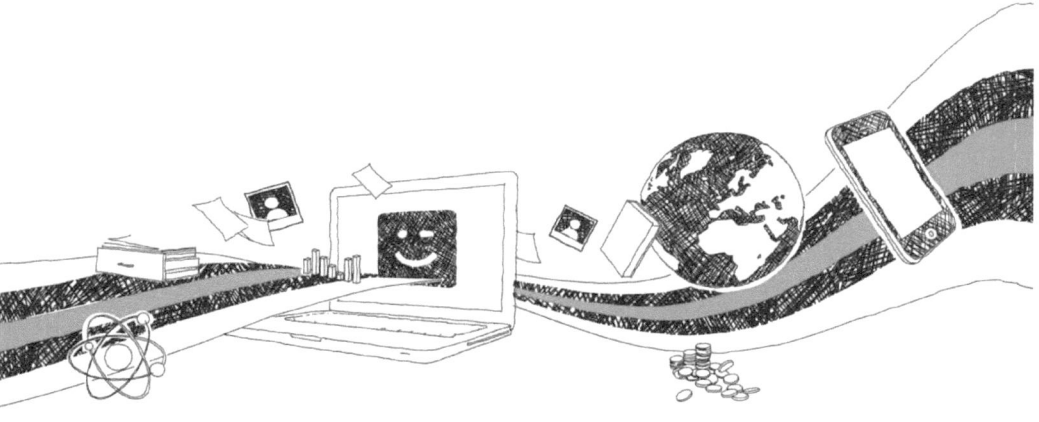

- We will publish your bachelor's and
  master's thesis, essays and papers

- Your own eBook and book -
  sold worldwide in all relevant shops

- Earn money with each sale

Upload your text at www.GRIN.com
and publish for free

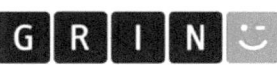